From A Man's POV:

How To Get A Better Shape As A Woman.

(Even If You've Been Overweight All Your Life)

By

William T. Walker

Disclaimer

Table of Contents

Disclaimer

Table of Contents

Introduction

Chapter 1: Adopting a Broken Fasting Regimen
What is broken fasting?
Weight reduction

Chapter 2: The Essence of Anti-inflammatory Foods

Chapter 3: Paying close attention to your macronutrients intake

Chapter 4: The Pros and Cons of the Galveston Eating Plan

Conclusion

A little note from the Author

Introduction
What's in it for me? Shed excess fat and combat midlife health issues.

I remember watching my helpless Sarah, literally living as a shadow of herself. I watched her put on the smiles on the outside like make-up, while she was cracking on the inside. I've always known my Sarah to be a strong woman, and somehow I had a feeling she was going to crack this also…

But, as time went by, she was getting worse, my Sarah was getting to yield point, and she became more hostile and I knew exactly what was going wrong with her.

A little hint; after our third child, Jason. Sarah at about the closing stages of her 30s, noticed she was getting bigger, of course, I wasn't seeing anything bad about that, but my Sarah wasn't in any way happy with herself, just as many other women out there.

I remember once catching my Sarah in front of her mirror, literally in tears picking up most of her nice clothes which would normally fit her perfectly, but at that time were nothing short of "too small"... By now, you should have guessed the problem my Sarah was struggling with; Sarah was overweight, and somehow she wasn't ready to accept it… (at least not in front of me!.)

I also suffered from this whole thing, as my Sarah became more hostile to me. But, I knew I wasn't ready to lose the love of my life, I set out seriously to find out anything, and everything that I could find, to help get my Sarah back in shape.

My journey to helping my Sarah recover has led me to uncover these three major steps that any woman out there (who has suffered or is suffering from what my Sarah suffered) can do and not only that, I will be sharing how you can start your journey to recovery as soon as tomorrow…

After, lots of research work, and reading and attending several seminars, particularly on health, I finally came up with these three major formulas, and I also noticed that it was very much recurring among many other success stories of women who have suffered from what was never their fault.

These three major formulas are the bedrock of the Galveston eating plan, formulated by Dr. Mary Claire Haver, and this eating plan is meant to get you over your midlife health crisis and prepare you to tackle the next phase of your life. My wife, Sarah is a major recipient of the procedures in this short guide, and I played the simple role of staying by her side through the journey of achieving better health and upgraded well-being.

In this short guide, we'll break down the three main components of the Galveston eating plan and explain how and why this method is so effective.

This short guide is designed to give you a straight-way, No BS approach to owning your body, and not living your life feeling like someone else.

If you're ready to start living your best life, let's dive right in, and see the basic steps you can undergo, to achieve the same goals and upgrade my wife has experienced.

Chapter 1: Adopting a Broken Fasting Regimen

If you are well-informed in the health and wellness world, the odds are you've reasonably heard a great deal about irregular fasting. What's more, even though it may very well seem like another trend diet from the beginning, it's an intriguing issue but understandably, the fact remains that it works.

What is broken fasting?

Simply put, broken fasting the name implies, is a diet plan that involves eating and fasting at different times throughout the day. Rather than zeroing in on what you eat, the irregular fasting diet plan is more about when you eat. Irregular fasting limits your eating to a characterized time. Recall, however, that no fasting timetable will compensate for a low-quality eating regimen. Regardless of what feast timing design you follow, make certain to have nutritious food varieties to give your body the fuel it needs.

Taking extended breaks from eating can be a sign of intermittent fasting, which may lead to a reduction in calorie intake.

Over time, losing weight can be made easier by eating fewer calories throughout the day. Studies recommend that irregular fasting helps decline calorie consumption, yet in addition prompts a ketogenic state which requires the body to utilize more energy, prompting more noteworthy calories consumed.

The uplifting news is there's no holy grail method for carrying out irregular fasting in your life. A lot of fasting styles are out there for your picking. Think about your lifestyle and decide which style is best for you as you learn about each one. Finding a framework that is functional and fits flawlessly into your life is critical to remaining steady.

At its center, irregular fasting includes adhering to a particular timetable of eating and fasting. Integrating it into your weight reduction venture is a useful practice because of its various medical advantages.

This is especially valid for ladies encountering hormonal changes during midlife.

A recent report showed that people who follow an irregular fasting plan for three to 24 weeks can hope to see a three to eight percent decrease in weight and a four to seven percent decline in their midsection size and that was exactly what Sarah experienced.

One more review led in 2018 uncovered that people with type 2 diabetes had the option to quit taking their diabetes drug in the wake of rehearsing irregular fasting for a year. Also, discontinuous fasting has been displayed to make other gainful impacts, like diminishing aggravation, bringing down the gamble of disease and dementia, and further developing temperament and mental capability.

The Galveston eating plan suggests integrating the 16:8 discontinuous fasting strategy. You would remain without food for 16 hours in a row, and eat within the eight hours left. Normally, the eating window begins around early afternoon when you eat and finishes at 8 p.m. at the point when you finish supper.

There are two reasons why this schedule is the easiest to keep up with;

One, it intently looks like the vast majority's normal eating plans, so you won't feel an emotional change.

Additionally, you won't feel hungry and won't be tempted to eat an unhealthy snack because you won't be awake for the majority of your fasting period.

It's fine if you don't enjoy eating during the noon to 8 p.m. window. Finding your ideal eating plan is everything. Depending on your schedule, you can change when you eat and fast, whether that means eating earlier in the morning or later at night.

Assuming the 16:8 example feels excessively prohibitive, you can continuously explore different avenues regarding the 14:10 technique or different varieties until you figure out your perfect balance.

It's likewise essential to slip into irregular fasting, particularly assuming you've never gotten it done.

Rather than making a plunge directly into it and skipping breakfast completely, take a stab at dunking your toes in first by step by step pushing back your eating time by thirty minutes.

For example, assuming you for the most part eat at 8, begin eating at 8:30. Increase this gradually until you reach your desired start time.

A great number of individuals who attempt to change to discontinuous fasting don't understand a chunk of time must pass to adjust.

At first, you may feel hungry and irritable (my wife frequently complained about this!), but be that as it may, those secondary effects ordinarily vanish soon.

Irregular fasting may not work for everybody's day-to-day plan, particularly individuals who have strange or long working hours or very dynamic ways of life that require eating all the more much of the time. In addition, research proposing that prohibitive eating less junk food (of any sort) prompts long-haul, fruitful weight reduction is rather conflicting.

Nevertheless, following a tough eating plan like broken fasting may increase one's likelihood of nurturing a dietary issue.

The significant advantages of broken fasting can be summed up under the following;

Weight reduction
One of the top reasons individuals take on another eating regimen is to get more fit, and some accept discontinuous fasting might assist with this. A deliberate survey and meta-examination in 2018 analyzed whether various types of irregular fasting bring about weight reduction. The exploration included six examinations going in span from three months to a year. Continuous energy restriction was used as a comparator intervention in four of these studies, which meant that participants consumed fewer calories than usual throughout the day.

Two investigations incorporated a no-treatment control intercession, implying that the benchmark group didn't change their dietary patterns by any stretch of the research.

Altogether, the impacts of irregular fasting on body weight were surveyed on 400 overweight and hefty people. The specialists inferred that irregular energy limitation was more successful than no treatment for weight reduction.

There was no distinction in weight reduction between irregular energy limitation and constant energy limitation. These outcomes depend on a few investigations, and more examinations are expected to affirm the impact of irregular fasting on weight reduction.

A later report inspected the effect of substitute day fasting (for example, eating as much as wanted every other day and nothing in the middle between) on calorie admission among 60 overweight people.

After a month of close monitoring, scientists found that while fasting on substitute days, subjects ate 37% fewer calories than they were used to eating before the review and shed very nearly eight pounds of body weight by and large.

While these outcomes might sound promising, the commitment to fasting should be accompanied by some significant counsel. That's why scientists emphasize that grown-ups who are well-advanced in age shouldn't perform fasting without meeting with their physicians to preclude unfavorable impacts because of basic ailments.

However, in this review, it is noted that a healthy and adjusted eating plan is logically vital to cultivate the helpful impacts brought about by substitute day fasting."

Overall health has also been mentioned as a potential advantage of intermittent fasting, in addition to body weight.

In another survey, various kinds of irregular fasting regimens and their potential medical advantages and related physiological components were analyzed.

The results of interest were changes in weight and metabolic boundaries (for example blood glucose levels and absolute cholesterol) related to type 2 diabetes, cardiovascular sickness, and disease.

About 16 human examinations were involved in the audit, and the larger part selected less than 50 members for brief timeframes.

The creators of this survey found that irregular fasting might be a powerful method for working on metabolic well-being for individuals who can endure not eating for expanded time intervals.

However, they concluded on the note that; "Embracing a normal, irregular fasting routine is a practical and economical populace-based procedure for advancing metabolic well-being."

Body Size
Our body size has an impact on our well-being. For instance, over-the-top fat mass adds to chronic weakness, and slender mass like skeletal muscle improves the well-being of individuals. A study involving examinations done on discontinuous fasting projects to decide their viability at further developing body arrangements related to sickness.

It evaluated three kinds of fasting regimens: Substitute-day fasting, Entire-day fasting, and Time-limited eating.

Substitute-day fasting regimen; which is between 3 to 12 weeks in length is really helpful at decreasing body weight, increasing muscle to fat ratio, reducing cholesterol, and fatty substances in typical weight, overweight, and corpulent people.

Entire-day fasting regimen; which is between 12 to 24 weeks likewise decreased body weight and muscle-to-fat ratio and further developed blood lipids (complete cholesterol and fatty substances).

Time-limited fasting routine; however, research on time-limited fasting routine was viewed as restricted, and clear ends couldn't be made. These examinations were restricted in span and size.

Longer, more powerful investigations are expected to decide whether discontinuous fasting is a successful method for further developing body synthesis and biomarkers related to well-being.

Chapter 2: The Essence of Anti-inflammatory Foods

Have you at any point felt like something simply isn't right with your body, but you can't exactly place what it is? As it turns out, you might be experiencing chronic inflammation, which has the potential to result in serious health issues in the future. What's more is that it adds to probably the most well-known and perilous illnesses in the US, like type 2 diabetes milletus, joint pain, cardiovascular issues, and Alzheimer's sickness. Irritation in the body can both stem from and fuel an expansive scope of conditions and illnesses, for example, coronary illness and joint inflammation, large numbers of which are related to the ongoing torment.

You can reduce the likelihood of experiencing related pain by consuming fewer foods that stimulate inflammation and more foods that reduce the body's inflammatory responses.
A decrease in estrogen levels is linked to an increase in chronic inflammation in women in their midlife stage. Such hormonal variances can likewise prompt weight gain, which further diminishes irritation.

At the point when you join these two elements with the regular American eating routine, which is high in support of a great number of food varieties, the scope of medical conditions might not be too far off.
The arrangement of this second part of is straightforward: stay away from high-incendiary food sources and integrate more non-inflammatory choices into your day-to-day dinners.

The absolute food varieties to avoid are; cheap fast foods, vegetable oils, and broiled foods. Omega-6 fats, which cause inflammation and raise bad cholesterol, are present in all of these. Anything with added sugar and counterfeit additives is likewise off-limits. Added sugar alludes to sugars that are added to food varieties, like table sugar, sucrose, and corn syrup. Saturated fat-containing foods should also be removed from your shopping list. This incorporates greasy hamburger, and cheddar.
At this point, you're likely considering what you are permitted to eat.

You still have a lot of options available to you, so don't worry. The main on the rundown is sound fats. Indeed, believe it or not: **FATS**. They improve brain and blood vessel health, regulate blood sugar, and reduce the risk of heart attacks, contrary to popular belief. Avocados, walnuts, olives, coconut flour, and sesame oil all contain beneficial fats.

Another must-have is also protein. It plays an essential part in bone well-being and keeps you full and filled after dinners. Anchovies and wild-got salmon are incredible choices for fish darlings, while chicken, eggs, and lean cuts of hamburger are great decisions for meat eaters. There's likewise protein in vegetables, tofu, almond milk, and curds.

Aside from sound fats and protein, starches ought to be a staple in your eating regimen. They get rid of unwanted estrogen while also providing your body with antioxidants and fiber.

Leafy green vegetables and a variety of fruits, such as; apples and bananas, are good sources of the type of carbohydrates known as complex carbs.

You would likewise need to add supplements for fiber, vitamin D, and omega-3 to your rundown. Albeit a few food varieties contain these supplements, you will frequently struggle with meeting the expected everyday sum from your dinners alone. Supplements for your diet can fill that gap and give you the amount of food you need.

What's more, we should not neglect water. As suggested by all well-being experts, make a point to get something like eight cups of water day to day. It is not required to be regular water at all times. You can add organic vegetables, fruits, or herbs of your choice to spice it up. Whole, nutrient-dense foods are emphasized in an anti-inflammatory diet, such as:
- Brilliantly coloured leafy foods
- Entire grains, like oats and earthy-colored rice
- Lean protein sources, like vegetables and tofu
- Solid fat sources, for example, nuts, avocados, etc.

These food varieties give cell reinforcements, which help the body to fight things that are possibly harming atoms in the body that heighten up your chances of being exposed to specific sicknesses and will quite often spike irritation.

The omega-3 fats in slick fish, pecans, and flax seeds are known to bring down unwanted reactions.
Limit inflammatory foods like white flour, added sugars, deep-fried foods, fatty meats, and cheeses while you work out the foods you ought to incorporate into your diet. You ought to likewise keep away from any food varieties you don't like too well. Assuming you're gluten-intolerant, for instance, stay away from wheat, grain, and rye items.

A typical day of eating could look something like this:

Breakfast
The cereal finished off with berries and a sprinkle of unadulterated maple syrup.

Lunch

An enormous kale salad finished off with barbecued salmon, in addition to a moderate measure of oil and vinegar
An entire grain roll

Evening nibble

A small bunch of blended nuts or seeds

Supper

A barbecued bean and lentil patty served over earthy-colored rice.
Steamed veggies
Warmed apple cuts tidied with cinnamon for dessert
Here are examples of food varieties you need to keep away from because they offer more harm than good. Sadly, numerous food varieties containing a piece of the conventional Western eating regimen can cause irritation. While following a this eating plan, abstain from eating:
- Food varieties high in soaked fats (counting red meat, cheddar, and food varieties made with immersed fats and oils)
- Full-fat dairy (like cheddar and entire milk)

- Refined grains (food varieties made with white flour, similar to cakes, treats, bread and pasta)
- Refined sugars (food varieties made with natural sweetener or corn syrup, including treats, treats, cakes, pop and natural product juice)
- Refined food varieties (inexpensive food and bundled accommodation food sources, similar to treats, chips, and microwave suppers)
- Food varieties that are high in sodium (counting many soups and nibble food sources).

Keep in mind, that you may not promptly notice the well-being impacts of staying away from these food varieties. You have to remain consistent and disciplined to encounter the greatest advantages awaiting you.
While food sources, as listed as follows should be included in your eating routine and you ought to zero in on eating these food sources, for example,

- Wild-got fish
- Flavors like turmeric
- Natural olive oil
- Vegetables (hold back nothing of varieties on your plate)

- Garlic
- Pecans
- Seeds and nuts
- Organic products
- Beans
- Natural grains

Regardless of the battle against eating grains in the U.S. culture, we shouldn't avoid them totally from our eating regimen. Entire grains, particularly when they're of the old grain assortment, have numerous medical advantages.

Chapter 3: Paying close attention to your macronutrients intake

Moving into the third and final bedrock, which is the macronutrient intake. The three most important nutrients your body needs to work well throughout the day are protein, starches, and fat. They're not quite the same as micronutrients, which include nutrients and minerals, which are lesser building blocks when compared to these macronutrients.

Macronutrients make up most of all the calories of your feast, and no particular food substance contains in equivalent measures all of the three macronutrients at once. Also, consuming one supplement more the others can prompt chronic weakness results.

These three macronutrients are the three essential supplements you want to include in your eating plan: solid fats, protein, and starches. You'll follow these macros rather than calories as you would ordinarily do with other health improvement plans.

This is a significant stage in the Galveston eating plan since this is the way you shift your body's energy utilization from glucose to fat.

To comprehend this better, how about we examine the study of digestion? At the point when you eat, your body scans the nourishment for carbs and consumes them for energy. After those are gone, your body naturally goes ahead to make use of fat for fuel.

Sadly, overabundant carb utilization can be tricky because it keeps your body from utilizing fat as an energy source. Also, the abundance of carbs can prompt the stockpiling of muscle-to-fat ratio. You know the unsafe impacts of overabundance of weight.

These three essential macronutrients are as follows;

Proteins

They are the macronutrients that fuel tissue repair and maintenance, particularly in muscles.

They're likewise behind your cell recovery, and getting enough of them is vital to keeping a solid body framework.

Truth be told, the body contains a large number of proteins developed from nitrogen-based building blocks called amino acids. Every gram of protein contains about four calories.

Nutritionists and diet specialists frequently prescribe getting 10% to 35% of your day-to-day calories from protein sources. Food varieties like meat, eggs, tofu, beans, and nuts are incredible protein sources.

Carbs

Carbs incorporate sugar, starch, and fiber, and they're the body's essential energy source. Your body changes over carbs to glucose, which powers the basic cell processes that keep your mind sharp during the day.
White bread, for example, is a bad source of carbohydrates for some people, but there are healthier alternatives. A well-balanced diet is built on healthy carbs, which help you stay active throughout the day. In short - not all carbs are "terrible" carbs!

There are four calories in a single gram of carbs, and getting 45% to 65% of your day-to-day calories from carbs is a strong reach.

Food surplus in carbs incorporates more straightforward carbs like potatoes and rice, as well as more perplexing carbs like beans, entire grain oats, etc.

Fat

Fat assists your body with putting away energy over extensive stretches so you can continue onward for some time without food. Furthermore, fat safeguards your nerves, controls your chemicals, advances supplement ingestion, and assists you with dealing with your internal heat level.

For some, fats add flavor and taste to numerous dinners. Subsequently, fat has been erroneously labeled as being terrible for your well-being. In any case, many fats are essential for the sound physical process, however, some ought to without a doubt be eaten with some restraint. For instance, immersed fats ought to include all things considered 10% of your eating regimen. Conversely, solid fats are unsaturated and can improve your well-being. Fats contain nine calories for each gram, and an extraordinary objective admission range is 20% to 30%. Olive oil, avocado, fatty fish, and meat are all high-fat foods that are also high in healthy fats.

To comprehend this better, we should talk about the study of digestion. At the point when you eat, your body scans the nourishment for sugars and consumes them for energy.

After those are gone, your body consequently goes to muscle to fat ratio for fuel.

Unfortunately, because it prevents your body from using body fat as a source of energy, eating too many carbs can be harmful. Also, the abundance of carbs can prompt the stockpiling of weight. You know the destructive impacts of overabundant weight.

This is where following your macros proves to be useful. Rather than eating a carb-weighty eating routine, you want to get your carb consumption down to just 10%. Healthy fats account for 70% of your daily meals, while protein accounts for 20%.

Normally, your body will find an opportunity to change by this shift. Try not to hope to see monstrous changes in no time, as most times, many people require between a month to about three months to adjust to this new macronutrient proportion.

You could likewise encounter aftereffects like sickness, exhaustion, and migraines in the beginning phases.

These are side effects of starch withdrawal, and they're typical for individuals who have been consuming diets low on carbs for quite a while. Some of the side effects can be reduced by drinking a lot of water and eating foods high in electrolytes like avocados, nuts, and green vegetables.

Chapter 4: The Pros and Cons of the Galveston Eating Plan

The Galveston eating plan doesn't require you to strictly measure calories, which might turn out better for certain individuals. Also, the eating routine highlights assisting you with creating smart eating routines and exercise propensities that will put you in a good position over the long haul as opposed to the confining and crash-consuming less-calorie eating regimens.

However, if you're new to the 16:8 eating routine, you must understand that it might forestall late-evening eating or nibbling. On the other side, it might make certain individuals gorge during the window available for eating to forestall sensations of craving some other time when they shouldn't eat.

The Galveston eating plan has the following advantages;

- **Could aid in weight loss:** Might be powerful in assisting menopausal ladies with shedding stomach weight.
- **Advances good dieting:** Advances smart dieting by zeroing in on entire food varieties, non-dull veggies, and solid unsaturated fats.

- **No calorie counting:** Doesn't expect you to consider your calories as long as you adhere to the basic principles of the eating regimen.
- **Helps in battling irritation:** Due to the emphasis placed on foods high in antioxidants and anti-inflammatory properties, it may assist in reducing disease-causing inflammation.
- **Diminishes the danger of life illnesses:** May safeguard against way-of-life illnesses like corpulence, type II diabetes, and coronary illness.
- **Directs glucose:** May assist with diminishing instinctive fat, fasting insulin, and insulin obstruction, in this manner forestalling or overseeing type II diabetes

Presently, on the other side, the cons and the disadvantage;

- **Low in fiber:** Fiber, which is necessary for regular bowel movements and gut health, is typically absent from low-carb diets.
- **High in fat:** High-fat weight control plans might be unsatisfactory for individuals who as of now have elevated cholesterol levels.

- **Restrictive:** Since the eating routine limits carbs and fiber, many individuals might find it hard to follow long haul.
- **Not upheld by logical proof:** Albeit the eating regimen is acquiring prominence, no logical proof has demonstrated that it is viable for weight reduction.
- **Cost:** The expense of keeping up with the Galveston eating routine is high, which can be an element to consider if you are on a careful spending plan.

Conclusion

Depending on your aims and objectives, these three major formulas which also serve as the bedrock for the Galveston eating plan can work, and will help you achieve your desired body and health goals, provided you follow them strictly.

This eating plan is probably more valuable with regards to weight reduction than other eating routines, like the Mediterranean Eating regimen, whose essential objective is life span improvement instead of weight reduction. Since, the eating regimen depends on broken fasting as a center viewpoint - and broken fasting has been proven through different examinations to help with weight reduction and glucose guidelines - you can most likely anticipate a few enhancements in those areas.

In any case, because the eating routine is prohibitive, certain individuals may not find it supportable for a long time. When you go off the eating regimen, you're probably going to encounter excessive weight gain and an inversion to your past metabolic state.

Thus, Haver suggests embracing these eating plan as a way of life, you'll follow until the end of your life instead of viewing it as a transient arrangement or a convenient solution choice.

It's additionally worth of highlighting that, all discoveries connected with the Galveston eating plan so far have been . There has not been an enormous, long-haul clinical investigation of this eating example to gauge how compelling it very well may be for reducing side effects connected with menopause and perimenopause.

Now, I don't promise you drastic changes in the next two months, but you have to make up your mind to be ready to put in the work to see results, and most importantly you need to have someone to stand by you.
I stood by my Sarah, and with her resilience, she was able to lose 60 pounds in 7 months.
And she is very happy with herself, so it's a win-win for me.

A little note from the Author

I'm sure you enjoyed reading this and gained some tips on how to live healthier. Kindly, do well to drop a review and visit my store on Amazon to check out some of my other writings;

https://www.amazon.com/author/williamwalker_writes

Thanks.